Amal KORRIDA
Youssef BOUCHRITI
Saloua LAMTALI

Applied Research in Nursing and Health Techniques

Amal KORRIDA
Youssef BOUCHRITI
Saloua LAMTALI

Applied Research in Nursing and Health Techniques

ScienciaScripts

Imprint

Any brand names and product names mentioned in this book are subject to trademark, brand or patent protection and are trademarks or registered trademarks of their respective holders. The use of brand names, product names, common names, trade names, product descriptions etc. even without a particular marking in this work is in no way to be construed to mean that such names may be regarded as unrestricted in respect of trademark and brand protection legislation and could thus be used by anyone.

Cover image: www.ingimage.com

This book is a translation from the original published under ISBN 978-620-6-71236-7.

Publisher:
Sciencia Scripts
is a trademark of
Dodo Books Indian Ocean Ltd. and OmniScriptum S.R.L publishing group

120 High Road, East Finchley, London, N2 9ED, United Kingdom
Str. Armeneasca 28/1, office 1, Chisinau MD-2012, Republic of Moldova, Europe
Printed at: see last page
ISBN: 978-620-7-61621-3

PREAMBLE

This research methodology course will enable students of the Instituts Supérieurs des Professions Infirmières et Techniques de Santé (ISPITS), in their capacity as future professionals involved in improving the quality of healthcare and health services, to consider evidence and contribute to research projects:

• understand the main theoretical bases of scientific research in general and in particular nursing care and health techniques in particular,

• explain the value of research in promoting nursing science and quality care,

• analyse professional situations from a scientific perspective,

• translate unexplained facts into a research question/hypothesis, and

• describe the various stages in the scientific approach to applied research in the field of nursing and health technology.

At the same time, students will acquire the knowledge and skills needed to carry out empirical descriptive research (qualitative, quantitative or mixed) and to write a research protocol for a healthcare activity, as part of their end-of-study projects (PFE). Students are encouraged to play an active role in their learning by reflecting on their reading, the knowledge they have acquired and their own personal resources, so as to be able to construct and complete their EFPs, and also to participate in the consideration of evidence in their practices.

TABLE OF CONTENTS

CHAPTER I

RESEARCH AND KNOWLEDGE

I.1. Definitions

I.1.1. Research

It is a formal process of acquiring and creating knowledge and understanding, using structured and systematic means and tools to gather information in order to better understand or explain a phenomenon. According to Legendre (1993), scientific research is based on a set of activities aimed at discovering the logic, dynamics or coherence of data, with a view to providing an original and explicit response to a well-defined problem or contributing to the development of a field of knowledge. Scientific knowledge therefore refers to a generalised set of laws and theories to explain a phenomenon or behaviour of interest acquired using the scientific method. Laws are observed models of phenomena or behaviour, while theories are systematic explanations of these phenomena or behaviour.

Scientific research activities must be :

• **Objective:** carried out in a spirit of impartiality (neutrality, fairness, integrity, accuracy) with attention paid to one's own beliefs and prejudices, and in a constant effort to be faithful and honest to the object of study. Also, its design must allow the use of relatively objective measuring instruments, so that each observer or judge who assesses the performance is able to provide the same report.

• **Rigorous:** carried out with precision, accuracy and meticulousness.

• **Verifiable:** can be confirmed by other researchers reproducing the same conditions. similar.

• **Generalizable:** The information, data, results and conclusions drawn can be generalized to different regions, communities or populations.

Scientific research also follows a logical order, principles and rules according to a scientific approach which, overall, is characterised by three stages:

• Observation is the first stage in the scientific process, which consists of observing and select a fact and formulate it in the form of a question or issue.

• A hypothesis is a supposition or plausible answer to a research question that is awaiting confirmation or refutation. It attempts to explain a group of facts or to predict the appearance of new facts. A hypothesis is not a random suggestion about the occurrence of an event, but a clear statement about what we expect to obtain, observe, measure or observe.

• Experimentation (i.e. the empirical approach), which refers to the means and tools (protocols, parameters, methods, calculations, instruments, etc.) used to test and investigate the various hypotheses put forward, and thereby confirm or refute them.

I.1.2. Concept/model conceptual

A **concept is** a general, abstract idea, attributed to a category of objects with common characteristics and enabling knowledge to be organised. The concept :

• Summarises and categorises concrete (real or tangible) observations.

• Links abstract thought (which operates on perception but not on reality) and sensory experience.

A **conceptual model** designed for the nursing profession or nursing, for example, is an abstraction, conception or mental image that guides nursing practice, research, education and management. It identifies the central concepts that will be considered as its pillars, namely :

• The person who is the beneficiary of nursing care (i.e. the individual, the family community or population).

• Health, which refers to the state of physical, mental and social well-being experienced by the care recipient.

• Care is the nursing, technical or clinical actions and interventions that ensure the safety of the beneficiary and aim to maintain their health and well-being.

• The environment, which refers to the beneficiary's entourage (financial, material, etc.), (e.g. socio-political, cultural, spiritual or ecological) and the context of its nursing care.

The advantages of conceptual models are :

• Define a practice (e.g. nursing),

• Organising your thoughts,

• Structure to observe and interpret,

• Provide the means to stand out from other disciplines,

• Identify health problems in a rational way (i.e.: Cartesian, methodical and therefore based on reason, the mind and logic), and

• To provide a guide to the application of the care approach.

I.1.3. Discipline (speciality, branch, science or field)

A discipline is a branch of knowledge developed by a community of specialists who adhere to the same research practices. It is the academic speciality of a student or researcher.
There are scientific and literary disciplines, and others that fall somewhere in between.

Examples:
• Educational disciplines (primary, secondary, baccalaureate, master's, doctorate, etc.),

• Artistic disciplines (sculpture, architecture, graphic arts (including painting and drawing), as well as music, poetry, dance, film, theatre and literature,

• Scientific disciplines that are often classified into three categories:

- The formal or exact sciences, where the systems studied can describe reality or even be perfectly hypothetical universes with no known concrete application. Examples: computer science and mathematics

- The **natural or experimental sciences** that study the rules that govern the natural world (life, physics, the universe, etc.), using the scientific method and selecting the most relevant models to study and describe reality. Examples: biology, physics, epidemiology, chemistry, astronomy, geology, etc.

- **Humanities or social sciences** that study human systems. Examples: anthropology, economics, politics, philosophy, psychology, communication, etc.

These three groups make up the set of **basic sciences** that serve as a basis for the **applied sciences,** which are oriented towards the concrete, tangible and practical application of knowledge and skills, in particular engineering, medicine, education, etc.

Special case: Nursing

These are applied sciences derived from nursing research. They concern theoretical, practical, clinical, ethical and deontological knowledge produced from conceptual models for the nursing profession. Example: the currents of nursing thought (Cf: Florence Nightingale, Virginia Henderson, Martha Rogers, etc.).

I.1.4. Empiricism

It refers to a set of philosophical theories that make observation, data and experience/experimentation the origin of knowledge.

I.1.5. Theory

It is a homogeneous set of ideas, notions, principles, rules or hypotheses on a particular subject. It is derived from empirical evidence, real or otherwise, and is subject to verification and control by reasoning and criticism.

I.1.6. Paradigm

According to the philosopher Thomas Samuel Kuhn (1922-1996), a paradigm is a dominant framework or model of thought that conditions researchers' perceptions, beliefs and values, and consequently their ways of interpreting the world, its events and phenomena. Like theories, paradigms can also evolve over time, keeping pace with progress and contemporary trends.

I.1.7. Epistemology

It is the theory of knowledge or philosophical discipline that explains the meaning of work, knowledge and scientific knowledge. It aims to clarify the conception of the knowledge on which a research project is based.

I.2. Sources of knowledge acquisition and knowledge

I.2.1. Through intuition (intuitive knowledge)

Intuition consists of guessing, sensing, feeling, understanding and knowing someone or something immediately, without going through the stages of analysis, reasoning or reflection. For Immanuel Kant (1724-1804), intuition is a source of knowledge, and 'pure' intuition is an infallible source of knowledge, since absolute certainty springs from this source. For Jean-Paul Sartre (1905-1980), the only way to know is intuitively, a mode of instant understanding, without the conscious use of reasoning.

I.2.2. By tradition/culture/authority

Knowledge can be linked to a shared culture, authority or tradition, and is often transmitted through participation, example, training or mentoring.

I.2.3. Through personal and professional experience or habit

An individual's (researcher's) experience may derive from his or her routine, scientific, material or symbolic activities and practices, or it may relate to the knowledge and skills accumulated and acquired during a given phase of his or her existence.

I.2.4. By reasoning (logic)

It is a cognitive operation which presents a situation in a reflective way, and which, through a series of experiments, leads to one or more results. There are several types of reasoning:

• Inductive reasoning, which starts from a set of specific observations and leads to a general conclusion.

• Deductive reasoning, which starts from a general idea and deduces specific propositions or premises. In logic too, deduction is an **inference** leading from a general statement to a particular conclusion. Deduction therefore makes it possible to establish a conclusion from the **premises** or hypotheses at the beginning

.

Table 1: Comparison between deductive and inductive reasoning.

Approach or question	Deduction	Induction
Objective	Uses a top-down approach (from the general to the specific). existing theories.	Uses a bottom-up approach (from the specific to the general). Generate new knowledge and develop new theories.
Issues	Check the hypotheses.	Answer the research question.
Applications	Often used in quantitative research using statistical analysis.	Often used in qualitative research

Reasoning by analogy, which is based on similarities and comparisons between ideas, phenomena or situations before reaching a conclusion.

Reasoning by the absurd (or apagogy), which consists of asserting the truth of a suggestion by showing the falsity of its opposite. This type of reasoning imagines absurd situations for an idea in order to invalidate or exclude i t.

• Critical reasoning, which is used to reject an opposing opinion or point of view.

I.2.5. By convincing data/results (conclusive, logical, well-founded, obvious)

The practice of nursing is increasingly based on Evidence-Based Nursing, i.e. on evidence, evidence provided by critical thinking and nursing practice centred on scientific research, and aimed at providing quality care to patients.

Nursing practice based on scientific research and evidence is therefore characterised by :

• Incorporating the best results of contemporary research,

• Integrating clinical expertise into patient care and decision-making,

• Consideration of patients' values and preferences.

This kind of practice therefore makes it possible to improve care, its organisation, management and their teaching.

I.2.6. The heuristic or scientific approach to research :

Heuristics is the art of inventing, discovering, finding solutions and solving problems by limiting the alternatives and basing oneself on insufficient, less complete or less obvious knowledge.

I.2.7. Using the empirical method

It postulates that direct experience of a fact or event through the senses remains the only valid mode of knowledge. Although it is open to error, it is an important part of the scientific process.

I.2.8. By borrowing and integrating knowledge and sources of information from other contemporary disciplines and professions

These include biology, medicine, physics, pharmacology, chemistry, psychology, sociology, epidemiology and so on. These different areas of knowledge represent a considerable source of enrichment.

I.3. The role and importance of scientific research in the perpetual evolution of knowledge

The ultimate aim of scientific research is to create and develop knowledge in a particular field. Nursing and health technology research also seems to have the same aims, especially in terms of improving health services, defining the parameters and roles of the profession, and guiding and evaluating professional practice on the basis of evidence (Wietrich and Régnier 2005). Other factors influencing the development of nursing care and health techniques include

• The health needs expressed by the population,

• An ageing population,

• Advances in science and technology are placing new demands on care, in oncology, surgery, radiology, pharmacology, bioinformatics and so on,

• The evolution of society, its needs and its service requirements: healthcare community, prevention, home care, analysis laboratories, etc,

• Globalisation and the democratisation of information and communication systems (multimedia, ICTE, publications, Internet, etc.).

I.4. Relationship and link between practice, theory and research

In nursing and health techniques, theory, practice and research are intimately linked. Certainly, through research, the theories formulated and already in existence improve professional practice.

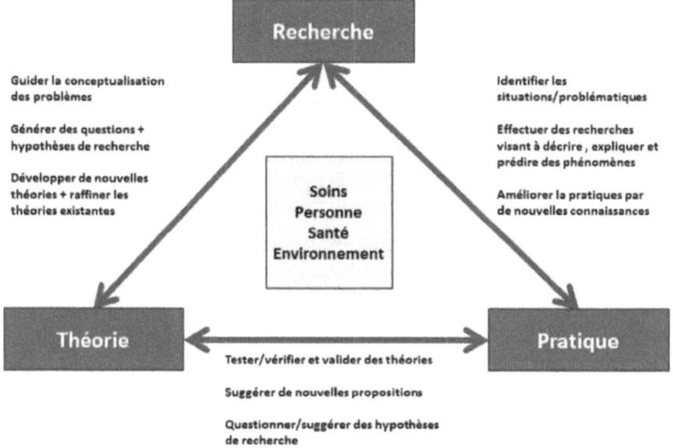

I.5. Special case: Areas of research in nursing

1. Clinical nursing research: This may take place in health establishments, hospitals, universities, outpatient clinics or community settings. It focuses on patients' clinical and health problems, nursing interventions and actions, and their evaluation (e.g. quality of care indicators, use of services: screening, consultations, hospitalisations, etc.).

2. Family nursing research: This most often takes place at community level and focuses on the patient/client, as well as on family issues such as care administration and childcare.

3. Nursing research based on occupational health: This takes place in professional contexts and aims to understand the impact of the environment and work on the health and well-being of workers, in addition to their nursing care needs.

I.6. Reflective approach/posture/practice

René Descartes (1596-1650) defined reflection as the action of the thinking mind. The reflective posture is therefore a mental posture that constructs the ideas that we develop and put into practice. It can give rise to thought experiments, as Newton (1643-1727) did with gravity, or Einstein (1879-1955) with the theory of relativity. According to Donald Schön (1930-1997), reflective practice consists of learning through and in action, i.e. supplementing academic training with training through practice, and also training through the analysis of one's own practice, during or after it (Vidalenc and Malric 2013). Reflecting on one's profession and practice requires mobilising a capacity for analysis, and involves examining one's actions (interventions, approaches, strategies, training), competences, skills, knowledge, attitudes, values, causes, successes, etc. (Lafortune 2006).

I.6.1. Aims of this posture

* Improve the effectiveness of your practice,

* Controlling your actions,

* Validate its practice and ensure its quality,

* Creating and generating new knowledge in relation to practice,

* Improve self-confidence and gain professional recognition (Jomas 2018).

I.6.2. Areas of application of this posture

* Medical and paramedical : nursing assistants nurses midwives doctors, speech therapists, etc,
* Social: educators, counsellors, guidance counsellors, etc,

* Educational: teachers, trainers, coaches, etc,

* Technical: technicians and engineers, etc.

CHAPTER II

RESEARCH METHODOLOGY

II.1. Types of research

Research can have several typologies and levels, depending on the different currents of thought, the nature of the research, its classification, and so on.

II.1.1. Depending on its use: Basic and applied research

II.1.1.1. Fundamental research (pure/theoretical research)

It focuses on the study of scientific principles, basic concepts, theories and laws in order to acquire knowledge, but not on their practical application.

II.1.1.2. Applied research

It is practical, non-systematic research that provides answers and solutions to specific questions in order to resolve a specific problem, whether societal, cultural, organisational or other. Examples of this type of research include :

• **Research and development (R&D)**: This often has an industrial or commercial purpose. For example, improving efficiency and innovation in the production of new processes, medicines, services or techniques, with the aim of satisfying the needs of a company's markets.

• **Research-evaluation:** Its aim is to examine and evaluate information about a particular research project in order to make the best decisions.

• **Action research:** also known as research-experimentation, is a scientific research process aimed at taking concrete action to tackle society's problems by steering it in the right direction.

II.1.2. Depending on its investigative tools and methods

II.1.2.1. Research quantitative

It is applied when the aim is to test, explain or evaluate a particular phenomenon or fact. It is characterised by research approaches that are generally deductive in nature and which aim to prove or disprove existing theories. It therefore involves determining and statistically measuring variables (or items) and testing the relationships between them, in order to reveal patterns, correlations or causal links. Researchers may employ linear methods of data collection and analysis, which result in statistical data. The underlying values of quantitative research are the neutrality, objectivity, and the acquisition of a wide range of knowledge about a considerable sample or study population (Leavy 2017).

II.1.2.2. Research qualitative

It is appropriate when the aim of the study is to describe, explore or explain a particular phenomenon or fact. It generally applies inductive approaches aimed at reinforcing certain understandings and knowledge and giving them meaning, especially in relation to events in social life. Qualitative research is often subjective since it is based solely on the experiences, stories, situations or lived experience of participants in a small, restricted sample. Examples:

- **Ethnography:** a field study developed in the field of ethnology, sociology and anthropology, consisting of studying the lifestyles of individuals, communities and populations in their contemporary and/or historical context.
- **Phenomenology: A** method of describing and understanding subjective phenomena, the experiences of individuals (e.g. quality of life, pain, satisfaction, etc.).
- **Grounded theory:** used in sociology to refer to the development of new theories based on data collected in the real world (Glaser & Strauss 1967).
- **Biography:** Refers to a story or account of a person's life.

II.1.2.3. Search mixed

As its name suggests, it employs both quantitative and qualitative approaches in the same study. It is commonly used in the behavioural sciences, applied social sciences and those aiming to bring about community change or social action.

II.1.3. According to its objective

II.1.3.1. Exploratory research

It is designed for new, poorly documented or undocumented phenomena and makes it possible to :

• Familiarise yourself with basic facts, situations and concerns,

• Formulate questions for future research,

• Generate new ideas or hypotheses.

II.1.3.2. Research descriptive

It is often used as a precursor to quantitative research models and consists of observing and describing in depth and detail a behaviour or phenomenon over a short period of time in order to describe the attributes (e.g. health determinants) in an objective and systematic way. It is often considered to be the most basic form of data analysis, since it identifies patterns in the various variables without going any further, i.e. in a purely descriptive way. The results of descriptive research are not produced to demonstrate causality or to give a definitive answer or to confirm a hypothesis. Various basic statistical calculations and analyses support descriptive studies, in particular prevalences, incidences, averages, frequencies, dispersion, confidence intervals ⁔ etc. Examples:

• **Cross-sectional survey :** Also known as a prevalence survey, this first level consists of estimating the frequencies and identifying the characteristics of a health problem, for example in individuals, groups or populations (Cf. p: 16).

• **Clinical case report** : Widely used in medicine and can be defined as a report or detailed account describing a rare, undocumented or unrecognised medical observation or information in one or more patients, in terms of laboratory tests, diagnosis, treatment, response to treatment, etc.

• **Case series** : **A** group of clinical case reports involving patients who have received a similar treatment or medical procedure.

II.1.3.3. Observational analytical epidemiological studies aimed at etiology

They include studies whose aim is to identify the causes of disease or the factors associated with health events, or to evaluate preventive or predictive actions. Whether on individuals or between groups (i.e. comparative), this type of analytical investigation is based on an observational and non-experimental aetiological approach, and includes :

• **Cross-sectional:** Which can, in this second level, formulate aetiological hypotheses comparing, at a short and precise point in time, the prevalences of a pathology in exposed and unexposed subjects, for example. Although the E+-M association between an exposure (E) or a risk and a disease (M) or a health event is often studied, cross-sectional studies cannot establish a cause-and-effect relationship.

• **Cohorts:** These are incidence surveys carried out either prospectively (collecting data over time) or retrospectively (collecting data in the past via patients' medical records or registers), by classifying patients into two groups according to their exposure status. Cohorts are followed over time to study the subjects who develop the disease in the exposed and unexposed groups (concept of relative risk RR). If cohort studies are repeated in the same people, they are referred to as longitudinal surveys.

• **Case control:** These are retrospective surveys involving two groups of participants: cases (or patients who are ill) and controls (those who are unaffected or not ill). Their aim is to compare the exposure of subjects to possible risk factors (concept of odds ratio or OR).

• **Ecological or correlational:** These are used when individual data are not available or when large-scale comparisons are required to study the effect of exposures on a disease at a population level. These studies are often subject to a type of confounding called ecological error or bias, which occurs when the associations between variables identified at group level do not represent those at individual level (Buckley et al. 2021). Example: time series.

II.1.3.4. Experimental analytical research (interventional or non-observational) for evaluative purposes

The aim of experimental studies is to determine the causality of an event or to measure the impact of a preventive, diagnostic, therapeutic, curative or rehabilitative treatment or intervention on biomedical or health-related outcomes. In this type of research, which complies strictly with research ethics, participants are randomly divided into a control group and an experimental group, which makes it easier to isolate the effect of an intervention. The experimental group receives the exposure/treatment, which may be an agent involved in the causation, prevention or treatment of a disease. The control group receives neither treatment nor placebo (a fictitious medical treatment with no pharmacological efficacy, in other words, no active ingredient). The groups are then monitored prospectively to identify those that develop the desired effect (Munnangi and Boktor 2023).

Examples:

• Randomised clinical trials (RCTs),

• Non-randomised clinical trials, for example.

Clinical trials are the most rigorous epidemiological approach for testing research hypotheses, and randomisation - the random allocation and drawing of participants into groups - helps to avoid confounding and minimise selection bias.

II.2. Different levels of research scientific

Post and Andrew (1982) distinguish 4 categories of research which make it possible to describe, explore, explain or predict factors, determinants or relationships according to each type of study.

Table 2: Levels of research according to Post and Andrew (1982)

Level	Question	Aim	Types of study
I	[illegible] [illegible] What are the factors?	[illegible] Name Describe Discover	Description and exploration factors Exploration Descriptive
II	Are there relationships between the factors? What factors are related to... ?	Describe the variables and relationships discovered	Discovery of possible relationships between factors or variables Description Survey Case study Correlational description
III	Explain the strength and direction of relationships union What is this?	relations	of associations between variables Correlational Explanation
IV	What is this? What happens if such a treatment is applied?	Predict a causal relationship Explain. Check	Testing causal hypotheses Experimental Quasi-experimental

II.3. Phases and stages of the research process or methodology scientific

II.3.1. Phase conceptual

The conceptualisation of research generally involves the following stages:

II.3.1.1. From the professional situation to choosing a theme for research

The researcher must ask questions by describing a professional experience, either during an internship, a field study, an irritation/curiosity, a major concern, an experience, a questioning based on theoretical or practical courses, readings, etc.). A good research theme must be well conceived and must satisfy certain criteria feasibility criteria :

• It must be achievable,

• It must relate to current health and social issues,

• It must be directly linked to the future nursing, technical, paramedical or other profession. biomedical research student,

• It must be original and its objectives clearly defined,

• Information and data must be available,

• The size of the study population or sample must be sufficient and well estimated,

• The deadline and deadlines for submitting the work must be respected,

• The study site must be easily accessible,

• Certain financial resources must be available to carry out the research, while remaining economical,

• Research leaders must be qualified, available and have a good scientific reputation,

• The research procedure and methodology must be well described and detailed,

• The researcher must frankly point out any flaws, gaps or obstacles encountered in the conceptual and/or other phases, and show their effects on the quality of the results,

• The analysis of the data must be sufficiently adequate to reveal its significance.

• Ethical considerations must be respected (integrity, confidentiality, authorisations, etc.),

• A good research proposal is also characterised by i t s   flexibility, adaptability, efficiency, etc.

II.3.1.2. Formulate a research problem (= initial question)

Once the theme has been chosen, the initial question can be formulated by asking questions about the situation in question:

• What do we want to show, study or understand when we carry out the study?

• What are the objectives and benefits of the study?

• What are the experiences and findings?

• What are the reasons for this choice?

The initial question is therefore a guide to progress in exploring and the orientation of the state-of-the-art phase or the bibliography of a research project.It must also be precise, clear and relevant, and could be refined throughout the work in order to properly target the study population and the focus of the work (Beziat et al. 2004).

II.3.1.3. Identify relevant literature = bibliography = exploratory phase (reading and/or interviews in the field) = state of the art

This phase includes reading, document analysis and exploratory interviews in the field.

(a) Literature and documentation

The tools used to collect data and documentary information may be
• Articles, publications, books, documents and study and expert reports,

• Theses and dissertations,

• Specialised encyclopaedias and dictionaries,

• Proceedings of conferences and scientific meetings,

• Press reviews or scientific journals,

• Specialist databases: Medline, Pubmed, Google Scholar, Clinicalkey, Science Direct, etc,

• Films, CDs and documentaries,

• Internet/intranet, etc.

(b) Exploratory interviews at

Interviews enable information to be gathered from people who can shed light on the relevance of the research. They are also useful in facilitating the exploration of aspects and measures to be taken into account in order to broaden or rectify the field of investigation, especially before committing major resources.

(c) Development of an exploratory interview (interview)

Exploratory interviews should be open and flexible, avoiding heavy-handed, numerous and overly precise questions. The aim is to listen to the interviewee in order to discover new ideas and avenues, to broaden the horizon, and not to validate the interviewer's own ideas.

(d) People interviewed

They may include :

• Patients,

• Users or staff of the healthcare system,

• Experts and professionals involved in the subject studied,

• Association staff, etc.

N.B.: Exploratory interviews are pre-tests and should not be confused with the "real" interviews or field surveys used during the methodological or data collection phase.

II.3.1.4. State the problem, objectives and/or hypotheses of research

The study's **problem** should lead to the central research question, after reformulating the initial questioning or the initial question.

The **objectives** are research elements formulated at the start of the study that will help to resolve the problem. They indicate the aim and the points to be reached once the study has been carried out, and serve to guide the research in its various directions and methodologies. In general, a project may have one main objective and/or several specific objectives. Research objectives must be feasible, clear and relevant. They are generally formulated using action verbs (explain, identify, study).

Hypotheses are assumptions or provisional answers to questions that have already been posed in response to a research problem (e.g. the occurrence of a health problem). As logical predictions, they are also based on existing knowledge, facts or evidence, such as experiments, theories, observations or previous studies. Hypotheses must be statistically tested and verified (see biostatistics course: null hypothesis and alternative hypothesis).

II.3.1.5. S. Development of a frame of reference (optional)

The reference framework is a body of knowledge, themes, concepts and legislative texts (charters, treaties, strategies, etc.) that are relevant to the theme or subject of the research. In other words, it represents the socio-economic aspect, the environment and the regulations in force.

II.3.2.Phase methodology

It is used to describe precisely, and in chronological order, the research protocol, in particular the data collection, the instruments and techniques implemented, the analysis and statistical processing of the data, in addition to the ethical aspect, in order to answer the questions and hypotheses formulated, and consequently to achieve the objectives and purpose of the investigation.

II.3.2.1. Definition of the type of study

The nature of the study in question should be specified: descriptive, exploratory, quantitative, qualitative, mixed, epidemiological (retrospective/prospective survey, case-control, cohort, etc.).

II.3.2.2. Description of the data collection process

The researcher is required to describe the data collection process in detail in the form of a **research specification**. This must contain the following information and criteria: The study population, the sample size, the cost and duration of the study/collection, the survey methods used, the administrative arrangements made, the resources and the logistics, etc.

II.3.2.3. Population and sampling

The researcher must define the population selected for the study, specifying the sample and calculating its size statistically. By definition, a **population** is a set of elements (human beings, living beings or objects) with a common set of characteristics. specific characteristics and subject to statistical study. The usual criteria used to define a population are geographical.

The **target population** refers to a study population from which investigations and generalisations are made. Clinical and demographic characteristics may define this type of population.

The **sample** refers to a subset of elements or subjects from the population under study. The size of the sample is determined partly by professional considerations and partly by statistical methods (Cf. p: 35).

Sampling is therefore the process by which the sample of a population is determined. The sample must be representative of the study population and of sufficient size to avoid selection bias. The different types of sampling will be described in detail in the third chapter.

II.3.2.4. Inclusion and exclusion criteria

They are criteria defined and determined before the start of a research project, with the aim of including or excluding certain characteristics and properties that are likely to distort the results and/or affect the homogeneity of the sample.

Exclusion criteria are conditions that exclude participants from a clinical trial or research study, such as age, gender, presence or absence of pathologies, physiological state, etc.

While **the inclusion criteria** set out the conditions for admission and treatment, the participation of subjects in a clinical trial or research study.

II.3.2.5. Methods and tools for collecting data

Once the research methods and paradigms have been chosen, the researcher describes the instruments and techniques that will be used in the study. These instruments provide qualitative information (interviews, observation, etc.) or quantitative information (surveys, questionnaires, measurement scores, etc.). The instruments used in field surveys include :

(a)Observation (often without being involved)

It is a qualitative process of developing knowledge about the person or patient, based on the observation of phenomena and facts about subjects or groups. The investigator examines and describes the information and events observed in a particular environment, without intending to change them.

Data collection tools: Global, focused, narrative and non-narrative observation grids participants.

(b) Interview or interview

It is a process that involves oral communication between two people: the interviewer and the interviewee. The interview survey is a conversation that takes place in a predefined context and is more or less directed by the interviewer, who must master this verbal exchange. The interviewee's confidence and the interviewer's benevolent neutrality are essential to the success of an interview. It can be used to :

• Gather information about the interviewee directly, including their knowledge, judgements, opinions, behaviour, beliefs, etc,

• uncover psychological processes and descriptive and qualitative data,

• test, confirm or refute the hypotheses of the study.

Data collection tools :

• Directed interview: Like the questionnaire, this consists of fixed questions. The interviewee responds in the form and at the time that suits him best.

• Semi-structured interview: This contains a number of open-ended or thematic questions designed to elicit the interviewee's opinion if he or she is reticent or does not respond spontaneously.

• Non-directive or free or open-ended interview: This contains a single general theme and/or a series of open-ended questions that correspond to the interviewer's instructions. The interviewee responds as he or she wishes, developing the aspects he or she wishes.

• Face-to-face interviews at work, at home, in hospital.

• Focus groups as a means of interviewing groups.

• Interviews using communication technologies: Facebook, telephone, Whatsapp, emails, etc. to avoid having to travel.

(c) Narrative or life story (autobiography)

It is a qualitative, intimate and non-analytical approach to the experiences of an individual or patient. It is therefore a veritable observatory of social life, from which people's interactions and actions are made and unmade (Le Breton 2004).

Data collection methods: Interviews or written biography.

(d) Questionnaire

A questionnaire is a series of standardised closed and/or open-ended questions in a generally quantitative survey, designed to standardise and facilitate data collection and surveys. The questionnaire survey is an often quantitative (sometimes mixed) method used in health science research (e.g. studies on pain, quality of life, knowledge, satisfaction, opinions, expectations, experiences, patient and carer behaviour, etc.). It can also be used to collect data according to certain socio-demographic or other variables (e.g. age, gender, place of residence, level of education, physical activity, etc.).

How it's used :

• is practical and economical (avoids travel, costs and charges),

• is not limited by time and adapts to the respondents' pace,

• minimises and blurs the effects of the interviewers' personalities,

• is designed and adapted to meet specific needs,

• makes it possible to work on a large scale.

Means of data collection: Questionnaires could be provided face-to-face, by telephone, via the internet (online), or in self-administered form.

Sidebar

For a quantitative research study, and during the methodological phase, it is also essential to define the :

1. Variables and indicators

The variable represents a measurable parameter or characteristic of the individual/sample/population such as: temperature, blood glucose, blood pressure, blood sedimentation rate, etc. (see dependent and independent variables, biostatistics course).

An indicator is a measurement, an element or an observed quantity that provides information about a phenomenon or field data. Example: Health indicators: mortality, morbidity, physical and mental well-being, etc.

2. Validity of a measuring instrument

The validity of a measuring instrument defines its ability to measure faithfully and accurately what it was designed to measure (for example: a blood pressure monitor, a questionnaire/interrogatory, a scanner, a screening test, an examination method, etc.).

Measuring instruments often contain margins of error due either to the healthcare professional (observer, operator), or to the measuring tool (which must always be calibrated), or to the person being examined or the object being measured (e.g. fluctuations in weight or blood pressure).

Generally speaking, the validity and reliability of an instrument depend on the types of error that occur. Two types of error can be cited:

1. Random errors that are not due to a particular cause are part of the reliability of a measurement of the data collected or of an instrument.

2. Systematic errors, which are due to a specific cause, are part of the validity of a measurement. They lead to measurement or information bias.

II.3.3.Presentation of the plan for processing and analysing the data collected

The researcher must cite the analysis instruments and tools he plans to use. will explain how :

• estimate, for quantitative data, the statistical relationships between variables in terms of mean, median, frequencies, contingency tables, X^2, value-, and so on. p, etc.

• it will process qualitative data: analysis of interviews, reports, newspaper articles, etc. press, strategic documents, etc.

Examples of statistical analysis tools: Excel, Sphinx, SAS, EpiInfo, SPSS, R, etc.

II.3.4.Fundamental ethical principles in research

Research ethics is a moral and philosophical reflection on the principles and standards that strictly guide scientific research from its conception, management, conduct, analysis, interpretation and dissemination. In the case of research on human beings, respect for the dignity and intrinsic values of individuals is paramount. According to the Belmont Report (1979), the basic principles relating to respect for human dignity are :

• Respect for the autonomy of subjects and protection of those whose

autonomy or **self-determination** (voluntary participation) is reduced, for example: prisoners, AIDS sufferers, children, or anyone with an illness, mental disability, etc.). One of the important mechanisms for respecting the autonomy of participants is the obligation to seek their **free, informed and ongoing consent**. Consent must be given voluntarily before the research begins, and participants may withdraw their consent at any time and request the removal of their data or human biological material (Canadian Tri- ouncil Policy Statement 2022).

• Concern for the well-being of research participants and their general quality of life, while protecting their **privacy** (opinions, place of residence, religion), **intimacy** (body, sexuality, relationships), decision-making capacity, **confidentiality** (information and personal details), safety, etc., and avoiding harm or discomfort (psychological, economic, legal, etc.) in connection with their participation in research investigations, and also maximising the benefits. (improved working conditions, promotion) and minimising the disadvantages (invalidity, disclosure of secrets) of such participation in research.

• **Fair and equitable** treatment of participants recruited for the research. The researcher must also honestly explain to the participants the nature and objectives of the research, as well as the means of disseminating and sharing the results. Ultimately, biomedical, clinical or experimental research involving human subjects must be evaluated and validated by **research ethics committees**, which ensure that research projects are carried out in accordance with scientific and ethical principles.

II.4. Phase empirical

II.4.1. Graphical presentation of results

Depending on the type of study and its hierarchical level, the data or results of the study may be presented using histograms, narrative text, photographs, tables, diagrams, charts, maps, figures or other means.

II.4.2. Interpretation / discussion of results

After presenting and analysing the data, the researcher must be able to discuss and explain the significance of the results generated, while referring to the objectives and hypotheses formulated at the outset (depending on the level of the study: achieved, refuted/confirmed) and comparing them with previous similar work. This approach will enable the researcher to make inferences, then conclusions and finally recommendations.

II.4.3. Conclusion

It is generally brief but concise and includes the following elements:

- a brief outline of the issues and objectives,

- he main results of the study,

- the theoretical contributions of the study,

- the limits of research,

- future research prospects or ideas.

II.4.4. Disseminating and communicating the results of research

Research findings and knowledge need to be communicated and shared with the general public and specialists for a number of reasons:

• Publishing the results of research means participating in the development of knowledge,

• Publishing research results maximises their impact,

• Publishing is also the means by which the researcher is recognised in the scientific community.

The fourth chapter looks at the tools used to communicate and publish scientific research.

CHAPTER III

SAMPLING

Sampling is an operation whose objective is to select a representative sample of the population studied. It is important to note that the results obtained on a sample are point values (exact values), whereas those relating to a population under study are presented by confidence intervals, which are parameters with a degree of confidence (generally 95%) fixed beforehand in the methods section of the research protocol. The aim of this section is to present the different sampling methods and techniques. There are two sampling methods: probabilistic (random) and non-probabilistic (non-random), and each method is made up of four techniques.

III.1. Probabilistic or random sampling methods

Individuals (elements or subjects) from the population under study are selected by chance. These individuals are then drawn at random, and will therefore have the same probability of being included in the sample. In other words, the sample will be representative of the population. There are four types of probability sampling.

III.1.1. Random sampling simple

The individuals in the population under study have the same probability of being selected in the sample. This technique involves randomly selecting a series of numbers (the desired number of individuals in the sample: sample size) from an enumerated list of individuals in the population under study, by drawing lots or using a random number table. On a list, individuals from 1 to 1000 are enumerated, and 100 are selected by drawing lots or using a random number table.

III.1.2. Random sampling stratified

Instead of selecting subjects individually from an enumerated list, these subjects are first distributed into groups or strata according to predefined characteristics. The number of individuals to be sampled per stratum is then chosen and finally selected by chance as a simple random sampling procedure.

III.1.2.1. Stratified random sampling proportional

The number of individuals to be sampled in each stratum is set according to a sampling fraction of 5 to 10%. For example, if we want to take a sample with a sampling fraction of 10% from a group of 300 students in the first year of ISPITS Agadir divided by options (or strata). For each option, 10% will be taken and the size of the sample selected by this method will be estimated at 30 students.

Table 3: Example of a proportional stratified random sampling method

Options	Workforce	Sample
Midwife	50	$= 50 \times 10\% = 5$
Mental health nurse	30	$= 30 \times 10\% = 3$
Laboratory technician	20	$= 20 \times 10\% = 2$
Anaesthesia and intensive care nurse	30	$= 30 \times 10\% = 3$
Multi-skilled nurse	90	$= 90 \times 10\% = 9$
Radiology	30	$= 30 \times 10\% = 3$
Physiotherapy	20	$= 20 \times 10\% = 2$
Social worker	30	$= 30 \times 10\% = 3$
Total	300	$= 300 \times 10\% = 30$

III.1.2.2. Non-proportional stratified random sampling

The number of individuals to be taken from each stratum is calculated according to its weight (or %) in relation to the total population. In the example above, the corresponding % is taken from each option. The sample size selected using this method is therefore 49.

Table 4: Example of a non-proportional stratified random sampling method

Options	Workforce	%	Sample
SF	50	$= 50 \times 100 / 300 = 16,67$	$= 50 \times 16,67\% = 8,33 \sim 8$
ISM	30	10,00	$= 30 \times 10\% = 3$
L	20	6,67	$= 20 \times 6,67\% = 1,33 \sim 1$
IAR	30	10,00	$= 30 \times 10\% = 3$
IP	90	30,00	$= 90 \times 30\% = 27$
R	30	10,00	$= 30 \times 10\% = 3$
K	20	6,67	$= 20 \times 6,67\% = 1,33 \sim 1$
AS	30	10,00	$= 30 \times 10\% = 3$
Total	300	100,00	49

III.1.3. Cluster or beam sampling

Groups of elements of a population are drawn at random instead of being chosen individually. For example, when studying a sample of ISPITS students in Morocco, a sample of one ISPITS is drawn at random from among the ISPITS in the country. Within these ISPITS, options will be chosen and within the options, the number of ISPITS will be randomly selected. of the desired students. The difficulty with this type of sampling lies in the constitution of thebunches.

III.1.4. Systematic sampling

The first element of the sample is chosen at random from an ordered list of elements of a population and, from this starting point, each element is chosen at a fixed interval (the sampling unit or step). For example, if the size of the population under study N = 1000 and the desired sample size is n = 100, then the sampling interval or step k = N / n = 1000 / 100 = 10; i.e. every 10ème elements on the list will be included in the sample from a randomly chosen number until n is reached.

III.2. Non-probabilistic or non-random sampling methods

Unlike probability sampling, the individuals in the population under study have different probabilities of being selected from the sample if a non-probability sampling method is adopted. There are four types of non-probability sampling:

III.2.1. Sampling for convenience or accidental

This type of sampling is adopted when it is easy to recruit individuals in terms of geographical, financial, informational and temporal accessibility. Two scenarios can be envisaged: (i) we fix n and the start of the subject recruitment period, then we recruit subjects from the start of the period until we obtain n (this date corresponds to the end of the period), or (ii) we fix the subject recruitment period, and we start recruiting subjects until the end of the period, the number of subjects recruited during this period corresponding to n.

III.2.2. Sampling by quotas

This type of sampling uses the same technique as non-proportional random sampling, the difference lying in the non-random choice of subjects in each stratum. This choice is made according to criteria pre-established in the methods section of the research protocol on the basis of a recent biographical review relating to the subject studied.

III.2.3. Sampling a priori or by choice reasoned

Based on a review of the literature on a topic chosen for the research, the criteria for inclusion and exclusion of individuals from the population studied in the sample are set. These criteria must be well documented, referenced and included in the If necessary, other parameters may be included in the measurement instrument depending on the specific characteristics of the population studied.

III.2.4. Network or snowball sampling

This technique concerns unknown or discrete populations made up of subjects who are difficult to identify or who have rare characteristics. The sample is built up from a small number of individuals who themselves recruit other individuals with the same characteristics from those around them (like a snowball that gets bigger as it rolls along). This type of sampling often uses tools based on social networks.

Table 5: Summary of sampling methods and techniques

Method	Technique	Content
Probabilistic or random sampling	Simple random	random each element of the population has a unique and opportunity to take part in the study
	Stratified random	sampling strata or subsets of the population are trained sampling sample is drawn at random
	Cluster or group sampling	Randomly select clusters made up of the population under study instead of individuals Systematic sampling Technique used when there is a ordered list of population elements
Non-probability or non-random sampling	Convenience or accidental sampling	Accessible groups
	Quota sampling	Extrapolation on the basis of certain characteristics
	Sampling a priori or by reasoned choice Network or snowball sampling	Choice of objects with typical characteristics Technique used to recruit hard-to-find objects using social networks

III.3. Choice of sampling method

The results of a study depend enormously on the sampling method; the sample must be as representative as possible of the population studied. This choice must be justified in the methodology adopted. For this reason, certain points must be taken into consideration, such as: (i) the nature of the study, (ii) the resources available to the researcher in terms of time and availability of data, and (iii) the degree of homogeneity of the population studied.

III.4. Choice of sample size

In the above, the sample size must be justified. This size depends on mainly on several parameters:

• The type of study: the size will be reduced for a qualitative study to respect the principle of saturation of responses. If, during a semi-structured interview, the researcher feels that the participants are formulating the same responses, then a smaller sample size can be used for fear of biasing the results. Generally speaking, for observational studies, it is preferable to have a sample size greater than 30.

• The nature of the population studied: when faced with a heterogeneous population, it is preferable to have a large sample (the size depends on the possibilities offered by each study, in particular the availability of data and easy access to participants).

• The statistical significance level: for applying certain statistical tests or for

To estimate certain parameters, it is necessary to have a large sample size.

III.5 Estimating the size of a sample

There are formulas for calculating the minimum sample size to obtain the desired precision. For example, the Slovin equation: $n = N / (1 + Ne^2)$ which is used when the degree of confidence cannot be specified, with :

n: size of the sample to be estimated.

N: size of the population studied.

e: margin of error in measuring the parameter to be estimated (e.g. estimating a % to within 5%).

Example:

If $N = 100,000$, and $e = 0.05$, then $n = 398$.

Other formulas valid under certain conditions for estimating n :

1. The sampling method chosen is random.

2. And the aim of the study is either to estimate an average based on a reference average (known) :

With :

$$n = V_x \times Z_a^{\,2} / d^2$$

Z_a : value corresponding to the degree of confidence (1 - a) according to the centred normal distribution reduced.

d: tolerated measurement error margin (often set at a / 2).

V_x : variance of the population studied. 1 - a: degree of confidence.

a: risk of error.

1 - a	80%	85%	90%	95%	99%
Za	1,28	1,44	1,65	1,96	2,58

3. Or to estimate a percentage based on a percentage of a reference population:

* If N is known :

$$n = \frac{Z^2 p(1-p)/d^2}{1+(Z^2 p(1-p)/Nd^2)}$$

With :

N: population size d: margin of error (2%)

p: proportion of the population

Z: value corresponding to the degree of confidence according to the centred reduced normal distribution.

$$* \text{ Si N est inconnue} : n = \frac{p \times (1-p) \times Z^2}{d^2}$$

* If p is unknown: p = 0.5 (50%):

$$n = \frac{Z^2}{4d^2}$$

CHAPTER IV

PUBLICATION OF SCIENTIFIC RESEARCH AND CRITICAL ANALYSIS OF ARTICLES

Research contributes to the production of useful knowledge that feeds into various disciplines. As a result, it is disseminated in a variety of ways.

IV.1. Research communication tools and publications scientific

IV.1.1. Oral communications

They include :

Conferences, congresses, seminars, symposiums, colloquia, meetings, open days, workshops, etc. Among the difficulties encountered in this type of oral communication:

• Limited presentation time (10 minutes for an oral presentation, and 25 to 30 minutes for a plenary lecture).

• Maintaining the interest of the audience: if there is a lack of enthusiasm, if the conference is   poorly chosen, if the environment is unfamiliar, if the people present are tired or distracted, etc.

• Lack of confidence on the part of the presenter, stage fright, stress, fear of being judged or of not getting the job done, etc. reflect a good image.

This type of communication and oral presentation could be transformed into written scientific documents such as conference reports, also known as proceedings.

IV.1.2. Written communications

Scientific writing can take several forms: paper (journal, book, thesis, PFE, poster or poster presentation, etc.) or electronic (electronic journals, virtual libraries, CDs, internet and intranet, etc.).

Written communications may include :

• **Internal literature**, including preliminary end-of-research reports, correspondence between researchers, research laboratory activity reports, etc.

• **Utilitarian literature**, including patent applications and popular literature such as scientific magazines aimed at a wide audience, etc.

• **Grey literature** consists of unpublished documents found in specialist libraries and information centres, including conference reports, patents, theses, dissertations (PFE) or reports, press releases, notes, etc. These reports can be read from three perspectives:

- That of the critic (representing the academic: teacher, jury),

- The researcher who wants to reproduce the study or use the same methods for other projects,

- That of the healthcare professional, programme manager for example, who wants to transfer the results to his or her practice.

• **Scientific journals** or **reviews**, which are serial publications that appear regularly (daily, weekly, monthly, annually, etc.), have a registered title and consist of a series of articles assessed by a reading committee on the basis of scientific criteria. The originality and scientific rigour of a publication are required by this type of scientific journal. Scientific journals are classified according to their fields of interest and their impact factors. The vast majority of journals are English-language. A distinction is made between "open access" journals, most of which charge a fee, and free journals, which often do not provide access to the full article once it has been published. The journals have guides with instructions for authors that should be followed when writing the article. The choice of journal is an important step, as it guarantees the acceptability and subsequent publication of the article.

• The **scientific article is** a type of scientific writing, based on simple investigation, the aim of which is to contribute to the progress of science or technology. It reports the results of a study designed to confirm or refute a working hypothesis. Once written, the article is submitted for publication to a peer-reviewed national or international journal.

IV.2. Types of articles scientific

There are different types of scientific article, each with its own objectives and structure. Here are the most common types:

IV.2.1. Original research papers

These articles present the results of new research, which may be of the following typesempirical, quantitative, qualitative, mixed or other. This type of article is also known as "original article" or research article, and generally follows the IMRaD structure (Introduction, Methods, Results, "and" Discussion) :

• **Introduction**: This section presents the context of the research, sets out the problem studied, and outlines the objectives of the study and its importance for the field of research concerned.

• **Methods**: This section describes in detail the methodology used to conduct the study. It includes information on study design, participants or samples, data collection instruments or procedures, and statistical analyses used.

• **Results**: This section presents the results of the study in a clear and concise manner. The results are generally accompanied by tables, graphs or other visual elements to illustrate the main findings.

• **Discussion**: This section interprets the results of the study, compares them with other relevant research, and discusses their implications. The authors may also address the limitations of the study and suggest avenues for future research.

• **Conclusion**: This section summarises the main findings of the study and highlights its importance for the field of research. The authors may also discuss the practical implications of their findings and propose recommendations.

In short, the aim of an original research article is to present new scientific findings, place them in the context of existing research, and discuss their implications for the field concerned.

IV.2.2. magazine articles

These articles examine, analyse and synthesise existing research on a specific subject. They offer a critical and constructive assessment of existing research in a given field, which classifies them as secondary-type articles. Literature reviews, particularly those of a systematic nature, are widely read and cited. This category of articles includes narrative reviews, systematic reviews and meta-analyses.

• **Narrative literature review**: This type of article is a narrative synthesis of existing studies on a particular subject. It focuses more on the narrative and qualitative analysis of the research. It offers a descriptive and interpretative perspective on the existing research on a given subject, emphasising contextualisation, subjective interpretation and selective selection of the studies included.

• **Systematic literature review**: This type of article is based on a standardised and rigorous method for summarising all existing research and data on a specific subject. It follows a precise and detailed methodological protocol describing the objectives, inclusion and exclusion criteria for the studies, and the research, evaluation and data synthesis methods. It adopts an exhaustive search of multiple bibliographic databases and a critical evaluation of the studies included, as well as a transparent synthesis of the results and particular attention to the management of bias.

• **Meta-analysis**: This is often combined with a systematic review. It is a powerful statistical synthesis used in research that brings together research data from various sources, especially systematic reviews, to draw more global or robust conclusions on a specific subject.

IV.2.3. Research articles experimental

These articles describe experiments carried out as part of scientific research, detailing the experimental protocols, the results and their interpretation.

IV.2.4. Research articles theory

They discuss concepts, models or theories, often without involving direct experimentation. These articles may contribute to the formulation of new hypotheses or research approaches.

IV.2.5. Articles from methodology

Methodology articles focus on the presentation of new research methods or tests or techniques, as well as the development of better versions of existing methods. These articles are important for the scientific community because they facilitate methodological progress.

IV.2.6. Short communications, letters to the editor

These are shorter articles that communicate preliminary results from original research or new and innovative ideas. They are often used to share important discoveries quickly. This type of article is particularly suitable for researchers whose results are influenced by time constraints, such as those who working in highly competitive or constantly evolving fields.

IV.2.7. Commentary articles or

They offer a personal or critical perspective on a specific research topic or field. They may also address ethical, political or social issues related to science. They are categorised as secondary literature and are usually succinct, around 2000 words in length. These articles do not follow the IMRAD structure. Each type of article has its own guidelines for writing and publication, and it is important to choose the appropriate type according to the content and objectives of each research project.

IV.3. Critical analysis of a article

Evidence-based practice (EBP) is based on the relevant use of the best available data from high-quality clinical studies in the day-to-day practice of healthcare staff. EBP therefore requires, in part, an ability on the part of healthcare professionals to read cutting-edge scientific articles, based in particular on a critical analysis of published studies in order to extract (or not) the data that can improve the decision-making process when dealing with patients. In addition, before embarking on an empirical study, the researcher is required to carry out a bibliographical search to establish the current state of research on the subject in question. This important phase in any research process guides the researcher in his or her own research and writing. A critical analysis of an article would enable the researcher to choose the best bibliographical references that would be useful. The critical analysis of a scientific article consists of objectively evaluating the strengths and weaknesses of a piece of research, examining its methodology, results, implications and contribution to the field of study. In the context of medical training, for example, it is the original article that is used for the critical reading o f an article (LCA).

IV.3.1. Key points to consider when carrying out a critical analysis of a article

• **The relevance** of the article to a given research topic must always be determined. The title, abstract and introduction should be examined to assess whether the study addresses a significant problem and answers important questions.

• **The quality of the methodology** used must also be assessed. The design of the study must be analysed, as well as the samples, experimental procedures, measurement instruments and statistical analyses. The strengths of the methodology should be identified.

• **The validity and reliability of the results** must be verified. The size of the sample, the measures used, the precision of the instruments and the robustness of the statistical analyses must be examined. The consistency of the results with the methodology and their support by solid evidence must also be verified.

• **The interpretation of the results** and the way in which they are discussed should be checked, as well as the justification of the conclusions by the data presented. Potential limitations or biases in the interpretation of results should be investigated.

• **The originality and contribution of** the article to the field of study.

• **The limitations and** practical or theoretical **implications** of the results must be assessed, and their relevance and potential impact discussed.

• **The clarity of the writing and the quality of** the article should be assessed. It should be also check the correct use of references and quotations.

It is important to bear in mind that the critical analysis must be based on objective evidence and arguments. The aim is to provide a balanced assessment of the article, highlighting both its strengths and weaknesses, and offering constructive comments to improve the research.

IV.3.2. Key stages in a critical analysis of a article

This paragraph sets out the questions that researchers should ask themselves to ascertain the key elements to be taken into account in a critical analysis of an article.The first step is to read the article carefully. To begin with, the article should be read in its entirety to familiarise yourself with its content, methodology and results. Taking notes during this reading is essential to remember the important points. Next, the objective of the study should be identified by clearly determining what the authors are trying to demonstrate or discover. This information is crucial for assessing whether the article achieves its objectives. Methodological evaluation involves examining the methodology used by the researchers to collect the data. Is it appropriate for answering the research question? Is the sample size adequate? Are the measuring instruments valid and reliable? And are the statistical methods used relevant? When analysing the results, the following questions should be asked: Are the conclusions supported by the data? Are the results consistent with the objectives of the study? Beware of unsupported assertions or over-generalisations. As for identifying the strengths and weaknesses of the article, the strengths may include a sound methodology, significant results and a relevant contribution to the field. Looking for what distinguishes this research from previous work and examining whether it contributes new knowledge or perspectives are also points to check. Weaknesses may include biased samples, undisclosed conflicts of interest or problems with study design.The final step is to check the bibliographical references. The references cited in the article should be consulted to assess the quality of the sources used by the authors. Are they relevant, up-to-date and recent? Are there any gaps in the literature review? It is also important to ensure that ideas are presented in a coherent and consistent manner. understandable, and that references and quotations are used correctly. The context in which the article was published must also be taken into account. Was it published in a reputable scientific journal? Has it been cited by other researchers in the field? It is important to take these factors into account when assessing the credibility and impact of the article.In conclusion, the critical analysis of a scientific article requires careful reading, an assessment of the methodology, the results, the discussion, the references and the overall context. The choice of article to read is important insofar as it provides useful information for the researcher's practice. The following diagram shows the practical approaches to critical reading developed by Salmi (2004).

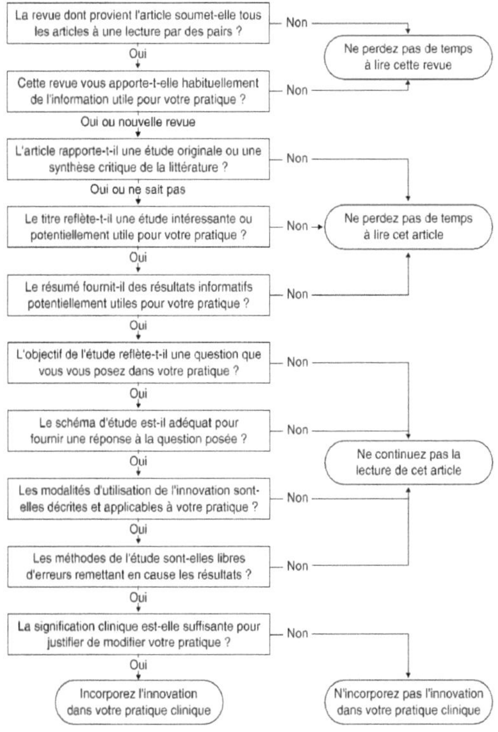

Figure 1 Étapes d'une démarche pratique de lecture critique.

IV.4. The IMRAD approach to writing and publishing a research protocol or PFE and its analogy with the conceptual, methodological and empirical phases.

Currently, the majority of scientific publications (articles, research reports, PFE/MFE, proceedings, etc.) are written according to the most widely used Anglo-Saxon method known as IMRAD: Introduction, Methods, Results, And or Analyses) and Discussion. This writing plan has several advantages: it makes it possible to create a document that is easy to read, logical, fluid, clear and universal in nature. Table 3 illustrates an analogy between the elements of the IMRAD plan and the conceptual, methodological and empirical phases mentioned in this research methodology course.

Table 6: Architecture of the classic research method and the IMRAD method

Conceptual phase	
From the professional situation to the choice of a research topic	
Formulation of the research problem	
Bibliography or literature review	I
Formulation of the problem and statement of objectives and/or hypotheses	
Development of a frame of reference	
Methodology phase (Research specifications)	
Definition of the type of study	
Definition of the population and the sample	
Choice of methods and instruments for data collection and analysis	M
Definition of variables	
Description of the data collection process Ethical considerations	
Empirical phase	
Presentation of results (tables and figures) Analysis	RAD
interpretation and discussion of results Conclusion (and outlook)	

IV.5. Intellectual property, Creative Commons licences and plagiarism

In academic and university culture, a new idea, concept or theory belongs to the person who created or conceived it. Usually, this type of creation can be protected by means of a trademark, patent, copyright, industrial design or circuit topography. This is **intellectual property** or **copyright** or **Copyright** © (equivalent to Trademark (= registered trademark) ™, or Registered Trademark (= registered trademark) ® in the industrial field). **Creative Commons (CC)** Licences are created to allow users and the public any exploitation of the works (which are protected by copyright), including sharing, distributing, copying, downloading, reusing, adapting, reproducing, by any means, in any format and under any licence, provided that cite the author of the original work in question.

Plagiarism is the act of appropriating someone else's ideas, words or products by passing them off as one's own (= without citing the source, references or intellectual property). It is a form of theft or literary/intellectual copy/paste = the fraudulent use of someone else's work either by borrowing or imitation. When sources are not mentioned, a designer's right of ownership is compromised. Plagiarism is intolerable and can compromise the reputation, credibility and image of researchers, as well as the higher education establishments with which they are affiliated (faculty, university, institute, etc.). To avoid plagiarism, you must mention the sources used and quote them faithfully (in the text and references (bibliography) when :

• borrowing ideas, concepts, documentation, images, tables, etc. figures, arguments, maps ـ etc.

• paraphrasing (rephrasing) or summarising ideas, a document, an article or a series of articles argues, etc.

CONCLUSION

Scientific research is a rigorous and dynamic process that makes it possible to examine, describe, understand, interpret, control, compare and predict phenomena or behaviour, and to create results and conclusions based on detailed studies, tests and experiments, enabling new knowledge and insights to be acquired.In the research process, methods and theory combine to create the research methodology. The methodology is the detailed plan of how the research will be carried out when different elements are provided. Beliefs or philosophical currents, in addition to ethical considerations, also influence the way in which a study is conducted. Although two studies may use the same research method (for example, a focus group, or a screening tool), the researchers' methodologies may be completely different, in terms of how they collect data, how they use these tools, their style of moderation, and the intervention and/or control of the investigator during focus group interviews.

REFERENCES

Beziat F, Cavrois S, Coatena D, Coilot MM, Donnet C, Haar I et al (2004). Le travail de fin d'études (TFE) en

soins infirmiers. Editions Estem, De Boeck Diffusions.

Buckley HL, Day NJ, Lear G, Case BS (2021). Changes in the analysis of temporal community dynamics data: a 29-year literature review. PeerJ, 9:e11250.

Cousi C (2023). The 13 types of scientific articles that can be published in peer-reviewed journals.

Scientific paper. https://methodorecherche.com/types-articles-scientifiques/.

Dabrion M (2012). L'analyse et le résumé d'un article de recherche, initiation à la démarche de recherche. Edition

de Boeck-Estem, 257P. ISBN: 978-2-84371-605-8.

Dartigues JF & Delva F (2009). A critical reading of articles: Analysis of the publication of a prognostic study 3/3. www.enseignementsup-recherche.gouv.fr/ressources-pedagogiques/notice/view/oai%253Acanal-u.fr%253A5311.

Fovet-Rabot C (2019). Writing a review paper, 7 points. Montpellier France: CIRAD. Frappé P (2018). Initiation à la recherche. Coedition Global Média Santé/CNGE productions. 2nd edition. ISBN: 978-2-919616-27-5.

Glaser B & Strauss A (1967). The Discovery of Grounded Theory: strategies for qualitative research. New York: Aldine Transaction.

Jomas P (2018). Helping student nurses acquire a reflective posture. Métiers de la petite enfance, 24 (264):12-14. Elsevier Masson SAS.

Lafortune L (2006). S'ouvrir à la diversité des élèves : Vers une équité sociopédagogique. 142 :86-88. Les Publications Québec français.

Lafortune L, Dury C (2012). Une démarche réflexive pour la formation en santé : un accompagnement socioconstructiviste.

Leavy P (2017). Research Design: Quantitative, Qualitative, Mixed Methods, Arts-Based, and Community-Based Participatory Research Approaches. The Guilford Press, New York.

Le Breton D (2004). L'interactionnisme symbolique, Paris, Presses Universitaires de France.

Legendre, R (1993). Dictionnaire actuel de l'éducation, Montréal, Guérin Éditeur.

Munnangi S & Boktor S W (2023). Epidemiology Of Study Design. StatPearls.

Post JE, Andrew PN (1982). Case research in corporation and society studies. Research in corporate social performance and policy. JAI press, 4:1-33.

Salmi LR (2004). Critical reading of a medical article: in search of genuinely useful innovations. EMC- Médecine 1(3):178-186.

Vidalenc I, Malric M (2013). What tools for a reflective approach in research activity? Revue Interrogations 16.

Wietrich L & Régnier JC (2005). L'initiation à la recherche en soins infirmiers. A tool for building identity
professional nursing. Recherche en soins infirmiers, 1{80):87-103.

The Belmont Report. Ethical Principles and Guidelines for the Protection of Human Subjects of Research (1979). The National Commission for the Protection of Human Subjects of Biomedical and Behavioral Research, USA.

Tri-Council Policy Statement: Ethical Conduct for Research Involving Humans (2022). Social Sciences and Humanities Research Council of Canada, Natural Sciences and Engineering Research Council of Canada, Canadian Institutes of Health Research.

Web Sites

http://www.ifsidijon.info/v2/wp-content/uploads/2017/06/2017-G%C3%A9n%C3%A9ralit%C3%A9-sur-la- research-en-soins-infirmers-.pdf.
http://www.prendresoin.org/wp-content/uploads/2013/05/La-recherche-en-soins-infirmiers-et-les- donne%CC%81es-probantes.pdf.
https://rrisiq.com/.

https://www.wikipedia.com/.

http://www.pearltrees.com/magoulou/propriete-intellectuelle/id5428587/item161179871#l829.

https://www.lib.sfu.ca/help/academic-integrity/le-plagiat.

https://fr.readkong.com/page/th-ories-de-soins-et-historique-de-la-profession-ide-4877578. https://actographie.files.wordpress.com/2013/10/type-de-publications-ipe.png.

http://reseauconceptuel.umontreal.ca/rid=1HZKGLHZ9-TYY7C4-82V/blt6060_c1_rexploratory_descriptive.cmap.

https://revue-interrogations.org/Quels-outils-pour-une-demarche,305.
https://cmapspublic3.ihmc.us/rid=1RPFL52Q3-23V4DC0-54Q/mod%C3%A8le_conceptuel_pourquoi.pdf.

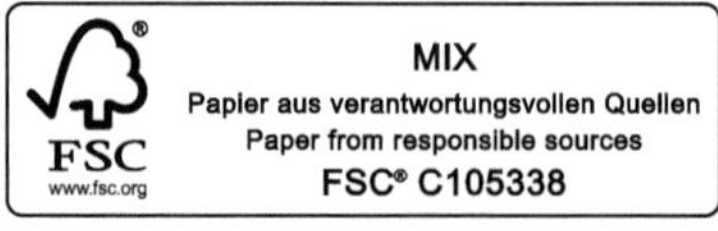

Printed by Books on Demand GmbH, Norderstedt / Germany